CONTENTS

INTRODUCTION

Welcome to the fascinating world of probiotics and the transformative power they hold in improving our health and well-being. In an era where our understanding of the intricate relationship between our bodies and the trillions of microbes living within us is rapidly expanding, the probiotic diet has emerged as a promising avenue for optimizing our overall wellness.

Our bodies are home to a vast ecosystem of microorganisms, collectively known as the microbiome, which plays a pivotal role in our digestion, immune function, and even our mental health. Within this intricate web of microorganisms, probiotics stand out as beneficial bacteria that can positively influence our microbiome and, consequently, our health.

In this book, we embark on a journey to explore the wonders of the probiotic diet and uncover its numerous benefits. We delve into the science behind probiotics, examining their origins, functions, and how they interact with our bodies. We also unravel the compelling research that demonstrates the powerful impact of probiotics on a range of health conditions, from gastrointestinal disorders to allergies, and from mood disorders to skin health.

But what exactly is a probiotic diet? How can we incorporate these beneficial bacteria into our daily lives to reap the maximum benefits? Throughout the pages of this book, we will unravel the answers to these questions and provide you with practical guidance on adopting a probiotic-rich lifestyle.

We will navigate the vast array of probiotic-rich foods, exploring fermented delights such as yogurt, kefir, sauerkraut, and kimchi, as well as the lesser-known treasures that can enrich our diet and nurture our microbiome. Furthermore, we will discuss the role of probiotic supplements and their potential benefits in supporting our overall health.

In our modern world, where processed foods, stress, and antibiotics have disrupted the delicate balance of our microbiome, it has become increasingly important to take proactive steps towards restoring harmony within our bodies. The probiotic diet offers a natural and holistic approach to achieving this balance, allowing us to harness the power of beneficial bacteria to optimize our health and well-being.

Whether you are seeking relief from digestive issues, looking to boost your immune system, or simply striving for a healthier lifestyle, this book will serve as your comprehensive guide to understanding and implementing the probiotic diet. By empowering yourself with knowledge and embracing the transformative potential of probiotics, you are taking a proactive step towards a happier, healthier you.

So, join us on this enlightening journey into the world of probiotics. Let us unlock the secrets of the microbiome together and embark on a path towards vibrant health, fueled by the remarkable benefits of a probiotic-rich diet. Your microbiome awaits its transformation, and a healthier, more fulfilling life lies just ahead

CHAPTER ONE

Introduction to the Probiotic Diet
Understanding the importance of gut health

Gut health plays a vital role in our overall well-being and has been gaining increasing attention in recent years. The gut, also known as the gastrointestinal tract, is home to trillions of microorganisms collectively known as the gut microbiota. These microbes include bacteria, viruses, fungi, and other microorganisms. The balance of these microbes in the gut is crucial for maintaining optimal health.

First and foremost, a healthy gut is essential for proper digestion and nutrient absorption. The gut microbiota helps break down complex carbohydrates, proteins, and fats that our body cannot digest on its own. They also produce enzymes that aid in the digestion process. Without a healthy gut, our body may struggle to extract nutrients from the food we eat, leading to various deficiencies.

Furthermore, the gut microbiota plays a crucial role in maintaining a robust immune system. Approximately 70% to 80% of the body's immune cells are located in the gut. The gut microbiota helps educate and regulate the immune system, ensuring it responds appropriately to harmful pathogens while avoiding unnecessary immune reactions, such as allergies or autoimmune disorders.

Another intriguing aspect of gut health is its influence on mental health and brain function. The gut and the brain are interconnected through a complex communication network known as the gut-brain axis. Emerging research suggests that imbalances in the gut microbiota may contribute to mental health disorders such as anxiety and depression. This connection highlights the importance of nurturing a healthy gut for overall psychological well-being.

Maintaining a healthy gut can also support a robust metabolism. Certain species of gut bacteria are involved in regulating energy balance and metabolism. An imbalance in these bacteria, known as dysbiosis, has been associated with metabolic disorders such as obesity and insulin resistance. By promoting a healthy gut, we can potentially support weight management and reduce the risk of metabolic diseases.

In summary, understanding the importance of gut health is crucial for maintaining overall well-being. A healthy gut promotes efficient digestion and nutrient absorption, supports a robust immune system, influences mental health, and plays a role in metabolic regulation. Nurturing our gut through a balanced diet and other lifestyle factors is essential for optimal health.

Exploring the benefits of a probiotic-rich diet

Probiotics are live microorganisms that provide health benefits when consumed in adequate amounts. They are commonly found in fermented foods such as yogurt, kefir, sauerkraut, and kimchi. Incorporating a probiotic-rich diet into our daily routine can offer numerous benefits for our health.

- Enhanced Digestive Health: Probiotics contribute to a healthy gut environment by promoting the growth of beneficial bacteria. They can help alleviate symptoms of digestive disorders such as bloating, gas, and constipation. Probiotics have been particularly effective in managing conditions like irritable bowel syndrome (IBS) and inflammatory bowel disease (IBD).

- Improved Immune Function: The gut microbiota plays a critical role in training and modulating our immune system. Probiotics stimulate the production of antibodies and enhance the activity of immune cells, strengthening our body's defenses against infections and diseases. Regular consumption of probiotics has been associated with a reduced risk of respiratory tract infections and gastrointestinal infections.
- Management of Antibiotic-Related Issues: Antibiotics, while essential for treating bacterial infections, can disrupt the balance of gut bacteria. This disruption often leads to antibiotic-associated diarrhea and other gastrointestinal issues. Taking probiotics during and after antibiotic treatment can help restore the gut microbiota balance and mitigate these side effects.
- Support for Mental Health: There is growing evidence suggesting a connection between the gut and the brain, known as the gut-brain axis. Probiotics may play a role in improving mood and reducing symptoms of anxiety and depression. While the exact mechanisms are still being explored, it is believed that probiotics influence the production of neurotransmitters and reduce inflammation in the brain.
- Enhanced Skin Health: The health of our skin is

closely linked to our gut health. Imbalances in the gut microbiota can contribute to skin conditions such as acne, eczema, and rosacea. Probiotics have shown promise in reducing inflammation and improving skin barrier function, leading to healthier and clearer skin.

- Potential Weight Management: Certain strains of probiotics have been associated with weight management and the prevention of obesity. They may help regulate appetite, increase the feeling of fullness, and reduce the absorption of dietary fat. However, more research is needed to fully understand the complex relationship between probiotics and weight management.

Incorporating a probiotic-rich diet can be achieved by consuming fermented foods or by taking probiotic supplements. However, it is important to note that not all probiotic strains are created equal, and their effectiveness can vary. Consulting a healthcare professional or a registered dietitian can help determine the most suitable probiotic strains and dosage for individual needs.

The link between probiotics and overall well-being

Probiotics, the beneficial microorganisms that reside in our gut, have been linked to various aspects of overall well-being. Their impact extends beyond digestive health and encompasses other areas such as immune function, mental health, and even cardiovascular health.

- Immune Function: Probiotics interact with the immune system in the gut and help regulate its response. They promote the production of antibodies and enhance the activity of immune cells, which can lead to improved overall immune function. A robust immune system is essential for fighting off infections and reducing the risk of autoimmune disorders.

- Mental Health: The gut-brain axis, the communication network between the gut and the brain, is a fascinating area of research. Probiotics can influence this axis by producing neurotransmitters and modulating the production of certain hormones. Studies have shown that probiotics may have a positive impact on symptoms of anxiety, depression, and stress.

- Cardiovascular Health: Certain strains of probiotics, such as Lactobacillus and Bifidobacterium, have been associated with improvements in cholesterol levels. They can help lower LDL cholesterol, often referred to as "bad" cholesterol, and increase HDL cholesterol, known as "good" cholesterol. Maintaining healthy cholesterol levels is crucial for cardiovascular health and can reduce the risk of heart disease.

- Allergies and Atopic Disorders: Probiotics have shown promise in reducing the risk of allergies and atopic disorders, particularly in children. They may help modulate the immune response and reduce the development of allergic reactions. However, more research is needed to fully understand the mechanisms behind this relationship.

- Digestive Health: Probiotics have long been recognized for their beneficial effects on digestive health. They can help restore the balance of gut bacteria, alleviate symptoms of digestive disorders, and improve overall gut function. Probiotics are commonly recommended for conditions such as irritable bowel syndrome (IBS), inflammatory bowel disease (IBD), and antibiotic-associated diarrhea.

- Oral Health: The oral cavity is another area where probiotics can have a positive impact. Certain strains of probiotics, such as Streptococcus salivarius, can help reduce the risk of dental caries (cavities) and periodontal (gum) disease. They can inhibit the growth of harmful bacteria in the mouth and promote a healthier oral microbiome.

It is important to note that while probiotics can offer potential benefits for overall well-being, they are not a panacea. Results can vary depending on the individual, the specific strain of probiotics used, and other factors such as dosage and duration of use. Incorporating probiotics into a well-rounded healthy lifestyle, including a balanced diet and regular exercise, is key to reaping the potential benefits they offer.

How the probiotic diet can support weight management

Maintaining a healthy weight is a common goal for many individuals, and incorporating a probiotic diet can be a supportive component of a weight management strategy. While probiotics alone are not a magic solution for weight loss, they can play a role in several ways:

- Appetite Regulation: Certain strains of probiotics have been shown to influence appetite and satiety. They can help regulate the release of hormones, such as ghrelin and leptin, which are involved in appetite control. By promoting feelings of fullness and reducing cravings, probiotics can contribute to better portion control and overall calorie intake.

- Energy Balance: The gut microbiota composition has been found to differ between individuals with obesity and those with a healthy weight. Imbalances in the gut microbiota, known as dysbiosis, can impact energy extraction from food and contribute to weight gain. Probiotics help restore a healthy balance of gut bacteria, potentially improving energy metabolism and reducing the risk of weight gain.
- Fat Metabolism: Some studies have suggested that certain strains of probiotics may influence the metabolism of dietary fat. They can potentially reduce the absorption of dietary fat in the gut, leading to lower calorie intake and promoting weight loss or weight maintenance.
- Inflammation and Metabolic Health: Chronic low-grade inflammation is often associated with obesity and metabolic disorders. Probiotics have shown promise in reducing inflammation markers in the body, which can have a positive impact on overall metabolic health. By mitigating inflammation, probiotics may help improve insulin sensitivity and reduce the risk of metabolic diseases.
- Gut Microbiota and Weight Regulation: The gut microbiota composition has been linked to weight regulation and adiposity (fat storage). Probiotics contribute to a healthy and diverse gut microbiota, potentially influencing weight management. While the specific mechanisms are

still being researched, it is believed that probiotics can alter the gut environment and affect the storage and utilization of fat.

It's important to note that probiotics are not a substitute for a balanced diet and exercise. They work best when incorporated into an overall healthy lifestyle that includes regular physical activity, a well-rounded diet, and appropriate portion control. Additionally, individual responses to probiotics may vary, so it's important to consult with a healthcare professional or registered dietitian before starting any dietary supplementation for weight management purposes.

In conclusion, while the probiotic diet alone may not guarantee weight loss, it can be a valuable component of a comprehensive weight management plan. Probiotics can help regulate appetite, influence energy balance, support fat metabolism, reduce inflammation, and contribute to a healthy gut microbiota, all of which can support overall weight management efforts.

The Science of Probiotics and Gut Microbiome
The role of gut microbiota in digestion and immunity

The gut microbiota, a complex community of microorganisms residing in our gastrointestinal tract, plays a crucial role in digestion and immunity. This diverse ecosystem consists of bacteria, viruses, fungi, and other microorganisms that work together to maintain a healthy gut environment.

- Digestion: The gut microbiota aids in the breakdown and fermentation of dietary components that our body cannot digest on its own. It helps break down complex carbohydrates, such as fiber, into short-chain fatty acids, which provide a source of energy for the cells lining the gut. Additionally, certain gut bacteria produce enzymes that assist in the digestion of proteins and fats. Without a balanced gut microbiota, our ability to digest and absorb nutrients from food may be compromised.

- Nutrient Absorption: The gut microbiota plays a role in nutrient absorption by facilitating the transport of certain nutrients across the intestinal barrier. For example, gut bacteria help metabolize and convert certain vitamins and minerals into forms that can be easily absorbed by our body. Additionally, they assist in the absorption of important compounds like phytonutrients and polyphenols, which have numerous health benefits.

- Immunity: The gut microbiota plays a critical role in educating and regulating our immune system. It acts as a barrier against harmful pathogens by competing for resources and space in the gut. Additionally, the gut microbiota helps train our immune system to recognize and respond appropriately to harmful invaders while maintaining tolerance to harmless substances. This interaction between the gut microbiota and the immune system is vital for overall immune function and protection against infections.

- Gut Barrier Function: The gut lining acts as a physical barrier, preventing harmful substances and pathogens from entering our bloodstream.

The gut microbiota helps maintain the integrity and function of this barrier by stimulating the production of mucin, a protective layer that lines the gut wall. Furthermore, certain gut bacteria produce short-chain fatty acids, which provide energy to the cells lining the gut and help strengthen the gut barrier.

Understanding different strains of probiotics

Probiotics are live microorganisms that, when consumed in adequate amounts, confer health benefits on the host. They come in various strains, each with its unique characteristics and potential benefits. Here are some commonly studied strains of probiotics and their associated benefits:

- Lactobacillus acidophilus: This strain is known for its ability to produce lactase, an enzyme that helps break down lactose, making it beneficial for individuals with lactose intolerance. It may also support digestive health and immune function.
- Bifidobacterium bifidum: Bifidobacterium bifidum is commonly found in the gut of breastfed infants and has been associated with the development of a healthy gut microbiota. It can help support the immune system and promote digestive health.
- Lactobacillus rhamnosus: This strain is known for its potential to support gastrointestinal health, particularly in managing diarrhea, including antibiotic-associated diarrhea and infectious diarrhea. It has also been studied for its impact on allergic conditions and may help alleviate

symptoms of eczema and hay fever.

- Saccharomyces boulardii: Unlike bacterial strains, Saccharomyces boulardii is a beneficial yeast that can help restore the balance of gut microbiota disrupted by antibiotics or infections. It has been extensively studied for its effectiveness in preventing and managing diarrhea, including Clostridium difficile-associated diarrhea.
- Streptococcus thermophilus: This strain is commonly used in the production of yogurt and fermented dairy products. It may help improve lactose digestion, support gut health, and contribute to the breakdown of certain carbohydrates.
- Bacillus coagulans: Bacillus coagulans is a spore-forming probiotic strain that is known for its ability to survive harsh stomach acid and reach the intestines alive. It has been studied for its potential benefits in supporting digestive health, immune function, and reducing symptoms of irritable bowel syndrome (IBS).

It's important to note that the benefits of specific probiotic strains can vary based on the individual and the specific health condition. The effectiveness of a probiotic strain may depend on factors such as dosage, viability, and the presence of other strains in the gut. Consulting with a healthcare professional or registered dietitian can help determine the most suitable probiotic strains for individual needs.

How probiotics influence the gut-brain axis

The gut-brain axis is a bidirectional communication

network between the gut and the brain, involving various pathways such as the nervous system, immune system, and hormonal signaling. Probiotics have been found to influence the gut-brain axis and potentially impact mental health and brain function in the following ways:

- Neurotransmitter Production: Probiotics can produce and modulate the production of neurotransmitters, chemical messengers that play a vital role in brain function and mood regulation. For example, certain strains of probiotics, such as Lactobacillus and Bifidobacterium, can produce gamma-aminobutyric acid (GABA), a neurotransmitter known for its calming effects. By influencing neurotransmitter production, probiotics may have a positive impact on anxiety, depression, and stress.
- Immune System Modulation: The gut microbiota plays a crucial role in educating and regulating the immune system, and probiotics can influence this process. By modulating the immune response in the gut, probiotics may indirectly impact brain function and mental health. Dysregulation of the immune system has been associated with conditions such as depression and neurodegenerative disorders.
- Inflammation Reduction: Chronic inflammation has been implicated in various mental health conditions, including depression and anxiety. Probiotics have shown potential in reducing systemic inflammation by modulating the gut microbiota composition and influencing immune responses. By mitigating inflammation,

probiotics may contribute to improved brain health.

- Gut Barrier Function: A healthy gut barrier is crucial for preventing harmful substances from crossing into the bloodstream. Disruption of the gut barrier has been linked to conditions such as leaky gut syndrome and neuroinflammation. Probiotics can support gut barrier function by promoting the production of mucin and strengthening the integrity of the gut lining. This can have a positive impact on the gut-brain axis, as a healthy gut barrier helps maintain overall gut health and reduces the risk of systemic inflammation.

- Vagus Nerve Signaling: The vagus nerve is a major nerve connecting the gut and the brain. It plays a significant role in transmitting signals and information between the two. Probiotics may influence vagus nerve signaling, potentially impacting brain function and mental well-being. This connection highlights the intricate relationship between the gut and the brain and how probiotics can influence this communication pathway.

The impact of lifestyle factors on gut health

In addition to incorporating probiotics into our diet, several lifestyle factors can have a significant impact on gut health. These factors include:

- Diet: A balanced and diverse diet that includes a variety of fruits, vegetables, whole grains, and lean proteins can promote a healthy gut microbiota. Fiber-rich foods, such as legumes, nuts, seeds, and whole grains, provide nourishment to beneficial gut bacteria. On the other hand, diets high in processed foods, added sugars, and unhealthy fats can negatively affect gut health by promoting the growth of harmful bacteria and contributing to inflammation.

- Physical Activity: Regular exercise has been associated with a more diverse gut microbiota and improved gut health. Physical activity can help stimulate gut motility, enhance blood flow to the gut, and promote a healthy gut environment. Engaging in both aerobic exercises and strength training can have positive effects on gut health.
- Stress Management: Chronic stress can disrupt the balance of the gut microbiota and impair gut function. Stress hormones can influence gut motility, permeability, and immune responses in the gut. Practicing stress management techniques, such as meditation, deep breathing exercises, and engaging in activities that promote relaxation, can help support a healthy gut.
- Sleep: Poor sleep quality and insufficient sleep have been associated with alterations in the gut microbiota composition and increased intestinal permeability. Adequate and restful sleep is essential for maintaining a healthy gut environment. Establishing a consistent sleep routine and creating a sleep-friendly environment can contribute to better gut health.
- Antibiotic Use: While antibiotics can be life-saving medications, they can also disrupt the balance of the gut microbiota by eliminating

both harmful and beneficial bacteria. Whenever possible, antibiotics should be used judiciously and only when necessary. If antibiotics are prescribed, it is important to discuss with the healthcare provider strategies to mitigate their impact on the gut microbiota, such as probiotic supplementation or post-antibiotic probiotic therapy.

By paying attention to these lifestyle factors, individuals can support a healthy gut microbiota, which in turn promotes optimal digestion, immune function, and overall well-being.

In conclusion, the gut microbiota plays a critical role in digestion, immunity, and overall health. Probiotics, with their diverse strains, can positively influence gut health, support the gut-brain axis, and potentially impact weight management. Incorporating a probiotic-rich diet, understanding different probiotic strains, and addressing lifestyle factors can all contribute to maintaining a healthy gut microbiota and reaping the potential benefits for our well-being.

Probiotic Foods: Your Gut's Best Friends
Fermented vegetables and their benefits

Fermented vegetables have gained popularity for their unique flavors and potential health benefits. Fermentation is a process in which microorganisms, such as bacteria or yeast, break down sugars and convert them into compounds like lactic acid, which act as natural preservatives. Some commonly consumed fermented vegetables include sauerkraut, kimchi, pickles, and fermented carrots. Here are some benefits of incorporating fermented vegetables into your diet:

- Improved Digestion: The fermentation process enhances the bioavailability and digestibility of nutrients present in vegetables. Fermented vegetables are rich in beneficial bacteria, enzymes, and organic acids that can support the breakdown and absorption of nutrients, promoting better digestion.
- Gut Health: Fermented vegetables are teeming with live bacteria or probiotics that can help restore and maintain a healthy balance of gut microbiota. The beneficial bacteria in fermented vegetables, such as lactobacilli and bifidobacteria, can contribute to a diverse and robust gut microbiota, which is essential for optimal digestive function and overall gut health.
- Enhanced Nutrient Profile: Fermentation can increase the availability of certain nutrients in vegetables and improve their nutritional value. For example, fermentation can increase the levels of certain vitamins, such as vitamin C and B vitamins, as well as enhance the antioxidant capacity of the vegetables.
- Immune Support: A significant portion of our immune system resides in the gut. The presence of beneficial bacteria in fermented vegetables can help support a healthy immune response. The probiotics and other compounds produced during fermentation can modulate immune function, potentially reducing the risk of infections and inflammatory conditions.
- Potential Weight Management Benefits: Some studies suggest that fermented vegetables may

have a positive impact on weight management. The beneficial bacteria and organic acids in fermented vegetables may influence metabolism, satiety, and the absorption of nutrients, potentially contributing to weight loss or weight maintenance.

Incorporating yogurt and kefir into your diet

Yogurt and kefir are popular fermented dairy products that provide a rich source of probiotics and can be easily incorporated into a balanced diet. Here's a closer look at the benefits of yogurt and kefir:

- Probiotic Power: Yogurt and kefir are known for their high content of beneficial bacteria, including strains like Lactobacillus and Bifidobacterium. These probiotics can help populate the gut with friendly bacteria, promoting gut health, digestion, and immune function.
- Digestive Health: The live bacteria in yogurt and kefir can aid in the digestion and absorption of nutrients. They can also help alleviate symptoms of lactose intolerance by assisting in the breakdown of lactose, the sugar present in dairy products.
- Calcium and Bone Health: Both yogurt and kefir are excellent sources of calcium, a mineral crucial for strong bones and teeth. Adequate calcium intake, along with vitamin D, is important for maintaining bone density and reducing the risk of osteoporosis.
- Protein Powerhouse: Yogurt and kefir are rich sources of high-quality protein. Protein

is essential for various functions in the body, including muscle repair and maintenance, hormone production, and immune support.

- Versatility: Yogurt and kefir are versatile and can be enjoyed in various ways. They can be eaten on their own, blended into smoothies, used as a base for dips and dressings, or added to baked goods for a probiotic boost.

Exploring the world of fermented beverages

Fermented beverages have a long history of consumption in various cultures worldwide. These beverages are created through the fermentation process, which converts sugars into alcohol or organic acids. Here are a few examples of fermented beverages and their potential benefits:

- Kombucha: Kombucha is a fermented tea beverage made from sweetened black or green tea. It is produced by fermenting the tea with a symbiotic culture of bacteria and yeast (SCOBY). Kombucha is known for its refreshing taste and potential health benefits, including improved digestion, increased energy levels, and immune support.
- Kefir Water: Kefir water, also known as water kefir, is a fermented drink made by fermenting sugar water with kefir grains. These grains contain a mixture of bacteria and yeast. Kefir water is a non-dairy alternative to traditional kefir and offers a tangy and slightly effervescent beverage. It is often flavored with fruits or herbs and is rich in probiotics, which can support gut health and overall well-being.
- Kvass: Kvass is a traditional fermented beverage

popular in Eastern European countries. It is typically made from fermented rye bread or other grains and has a slightly sour and tangy flavor. Kvass is known for its probiotic content and may offer digestive benefits, as well as potential antioxidant properties.

- Non-Dairy Fermented Drinks: In addition to dairy-based fermented beverages, there is a growing variety of non-dairy options available. Fermented drinks made from coconut water, almond milk, or other plant-based ingredients are becoming increasingly popular. These non-dairy options provide a range of flavors and probiotic benefits for those who avoid or prefer to limit dairy consumption.

Other probiotic-rich foods to add to your plate

Probiotics are not limited to fermented vegetables and dairy products. There are several other foods that can be incorporated into your diet to increase your probiotic intake. Here are some examples:

- Miso: Miso is a traditional Japanese paste made from fermented soybeans, rice, or barley. It is commonly used in soups, dressings, and marinades. Miso contains probiotic bacteria and is also a good source of essential minerals and antioxidants.
- Tempeh: Tempeh is a fermented soybean product originating from Indonesia. It has a firm texture and a nutty flavor. Tempeh is rich in probiotics, protein, fiber, and various nutrients. It can be used as a meat substitute in many dishes, making it a

popular choice for vegetarians and vegans.

- Natto: Natto is a traditional Japanese food made from fermented soybeans. It has a distinctive flavor and slimy texture. Natto is rich in a specific probiotic strain called Bacillus subtilis, which has been associated with various health benefits. It is often consumed with rice and other condiments.
- Kimchi: Kimchi, a staple in Korean cuisine, is a fermented vegetable dish made primarily from cabbage and radishes. It is seasoned with spices, garlic, and chili peppers. Kimchi is known for its tangy and spicy flavor and offers a range of beneficial bacteria. It is also a good source of vitamins A, C, and K, as well as antioxidants.
- Sour Pickles: Sour pickles are cucumbers that have been fermented in a brine solution. They are packed with probiotics and have a tangy and sour taste. It's important to choose naturally fermented pickles rather than those made with vinegar, as the latter do not provide the same probiotic benefits.

Incorporating these probiotic-rich foods into your diet can help diversify your gut microbiota and support overall gut health. Experimenting with different fermented foods and finding what suits your taste preferences can make it easier to enjoy the benefits of probiotics.

The Probiotic Diet Pyramid
Foundation: Whole grains and fiber for a healthy gut

The foundation of a healthy gut starts with a balanced and nutritious diet that includes whole grains and fiber-rich foods. Here's why they are essential for maintaining gut health:

- Whole Grains: Whole grains, such as oats, brown rice, quinoa, and whole wheat, are excellent sources of dietary fiber, vitamins, minerals, and antioxidants. These grains contain all parts of the grain, including the bran, germ, and endosperm, providing a wide range of nutrients. Whole grains are also rich in prebiotic fibers, which serve as food for the beneficial bacteria in the gut. By promoting the growth of good bacteria, whole grains contribute to a healthy gut microbiota and support digestion and regular bowel movements.
- Dietary Fiber: Fiber is a type of carbohydrate that cannot be digested by the human body. However, it plays a crucial role in maintaining a healthy gut. There are two types of fiber: soluble and insoluble. Soluble fiber absorbs water and forms a gel-like substance in the digestive tract, which helps soften the stool and supports healthy bowel movements. Insoluble fiber adds bulk to the stool, aiding in its movement through the digestive system. By including a variety of high-fiber foods in your diet, such as fruits, vegetables, legumes, and whole grains, you can promote regularity, prevent constipation, and support overall gut health.

Level 1: Probiotic fruits and vegetables

In addition to whole grains and fiber, incorporating probiotic-rich fruits and vegetables into your diet can further enhance gut health. These foods contain natural probiotics that can support a diverse and balanced gut microbiota. Here are some examples of probiotic fruits and vegetables:

- Fermented Sauerkraut: Sauerkraut is made from fermented cabbage and is rich in probiotics, including lactobacilli. It offers the benefits of both fiber and live beneficial bacteria, promoting digestive health and supporting a healthy gut microbiota.
- Fermented Pickles: Fermented pickles, made from cucumbers, are a tangy and probiotic-rich addition to your diet. They are low in calories and can provide beneficial bacteria for gut health. It's important to choose naturally fermented pickles rather than those made with vinegar, as the latter do not offer the same probiotic benefits.
- Kimchi: Kimchi, a staple in Korean cuisine, is a spicy fermented vegetable dish made primarily from cabbage and radishes. It contains a variety of probiotic bacteria strains, along with vitamins, minerals, and antioxidants. Kimchi can add flavor and probiotic benefits to your meals.
- Kefir: While kefir is commonly associated with dairy, there are also non-dairy options available, such as coconut kefir or water kefir. These fermented beverages are rich in probiotics and can be a suitable choice for those who avoid or limit dairy consumption. They offer a refreshing and probiotic-rich addition to your diet.

Level 2: Lean proteins and fermented dairy

To support gut health, it's important to include lean

proteins and fermented dairy products in your diet. These foods provide essential nutrients and can contribute to a healthy gut microbiota. Here's why they are beneficial:

- Lean Proteins: Lean proteins, such as skinless poultry, fish, tofu, and legumes, provide amino acids, which are the building blocks of proteins. These proteins are necessary for tissue repair, muscle synthesis, and the production of enzymes and hormones. Consuming adequate amounts of lean proteins can help maintain a healthy gut lining and support the growth of beneficial gut bacteria.

- Fermented Dairy: Fermented dairy products like yogurt and kefir are excellent sources of probiotics. They contain beneficial bacteria that can help restore and maintain a healthy gut microbiota. These dairy products also offer calcium, protein, and other essential nutrients. Opt for plain, unsweetened varieties to avoid added sugars and artificial flavors.

Level 3: Healthy fats and oils for gut nourishment

Including healthy fats and oils in your diet is crucial for gut nourishment and overall well-being. Here are some examples of healthy fats that can benefit your gut health:

- Extra Virgin Olive Oil: Extra virgin olive oil is rich in monounsaturated fats, which have been associated with numerous health benefits. It also contains polyphenols, which have antioxidant and anti-inflammatory properties. These components can contribute to a healthy gut environment and support gut health.

- Avocado: Avocado is a nutrient-dense fruit that provides healthy fats, including monounsaturated fats and omega-3 fatty acids. These fats are beneficial for the gut as they help reduce inflammation and promote proper nutrient absorption. Avocado also contains fiber, which supports digestive health.
- Nuts and Seeds: Nuts and seeds, such as almonds, walnuts, chia seeds, and flaxseeds, are excellent sources of healthy fats and fiber. They provide a range of nutrients, including omega-3 fatty acids and antioxidants. These fats and fibers can help nourish the gut and promote a healthy gut microbiota.
- Fatty Fish: Fatty fish, such as salmon, mackerel, and sardines, are rich in omega-3 fatty acids. These fats have anti-inflammatory properties and can help maintain a healthy gut lining. Omega-3 fatty acids also support overall heart health and brain function.

Incorporating these different levels into your diet can provide a holistic approach to promoting gut health. Whole grains and fiber provide the foundation, while probiotic fruits and vegetables, lean proteins, fermented dairy, and healthy fats nourish the gut and support a diverse gut microbiota. By combining these elements, you can create a well-rounded and gut-friendly eating plan.

Meal Planning on the Probiotic Diet
Designing balanced meals with probiotic components

When it comes to designing balanced meals with probiotic components, it's important to include a variety of nutrient-dense foods that promote gut health. Here's a guide to creating meals that incorporate probiotics:

- Start with a Base: Begin by choosing a base for your meal, such as whole grains, leafy greens, or a blend of vegetables. These provide essential nutrients, fiber, and a foundation for building a balanced plate.
- Add Probiotic Foods: Incorporate probiotic-rich foods into your meals to support gut health. This can include fermented vegetables like sauerkraut or kimchi, fermented dairy products like yogurt or kefir, or plant-based options like tempeh or miso. These probiotic components introduce beneficial bacteria into your gut, promoting a diverse microbiota.
- Include Lean Protein: To ensure satiety and provide essential amino acids, include a source of lean protein in your meal. This can include options such as grilled chicken, fish, tofu, or legumes. Lean protein helps support muscle growth, repair, and overall body function.
- Add Healthy Fats: Incorporate healthy fats into your meals for their beneficial properties. Avocado, nuts, seeds, and extra virgin olive oil are excellent choices. Healthy fats provide energy, support nutrient absorption, and help maintain the integrity of the gut lining.
- Incorporate Fiber-Rich Foods: To support digestion and promote a healthy gut, include fiber-rich foods in your meals. This can include whole grains, fruits, vegetables, and legumes. Fiber aids in maintaining regular bowel movements, feeds the beneficial bacteria in the

gut, and contributes to overall gut health.

- Opt for Colorful Produce: Include a variety of colorful fruits and vegetables in your meals to provide a wide range of vitamins, minerals, and antioxidants. These plant-based foods are not only nutrient-dense but also promote a healthy gut environment.

Probiotic breakfast ideas for a nutritious start

Breakfast is an ideal time to incorporate probiotics into your daily routine. Here are some probiotic-rich breakfast ideas to kickstart your day with a nutritious boost:

- Yogurt Parfait: Layer plain yogurt with fresh berries, a sprinkle of nuts or seeds, and a drizzle of honey. This simple and delicious breakfast provides probiotics from the yogurt and a range of nutrients from the fruits and nuts.
- Overnight Chia Pudding: Combine chia seeds with your choice of milk (dairy or plant-based) and a spoonful of yogurt. Let it sit in the refrigerator overnight to create a creamy pudding-like texture. Top with sliced fruits, a dollop of nut butter, or a sprinkle of granola for added flavor and nutrients.
- Smoothie Bowl: Blend together a combination of frozen fruits, spinach or kale, yogurt, and a liquid of your choice (such as almond milk or coconut water) to create a thick smoothie. Pour it into a bowl and top with probiotic-rich toppings like sliced banana, granola, and a drizzle of honey.
- Fermented Oats: Cook your oats with a twist by using fermented dairy or non-dairy yogurt instead of water or milk. This adds a tangy

flavor and introduces probiotics to your breakfast. Top with fresh fruits, nuts, and a sprinkle of cinnamon for added taste and nutrients.

Probiotic-packed lunches for sustained energy

Lunchtime is an opportunity to nourish your body with a probiotic-packed meal that will sustain your energy throughout the day. Here are some ideas for incorporating probiotics into your lunches:

- Buddha Bowl: Build a bowl with a variety of components, such as cooked quinoa or brown rice, roasted vegetables, sautéed greens, fermented kimchi or sauerkraut, and a protein source like grilled chicken, tofu, or chickpeas. Drizzle with a probiotic-rich dressing like tahini or yogurt-based dressing for added flavor.
- Wraps or Sandwiches: Fill whole grain wraps or bread with lean protein options like turkey, grilled salmon, or tempeh, along with probiotic-rich ingredients like sliced avocado, fermented pickles, sprouts, and a smear of probiotic-rich hummus or Greek yogurt spread.
- Grain Salads: Create a hearty salad with a base of cooked grains like quinoa or farro. Add in a mix of fresh vegetables, such as cucumbers, tomatoes, and bell peppers, and incorporate probiotic elements like crumbled feta cheese, olives, and a dressing made with yogurt and herbs.
- Sushi Rolls: Make your own sushi rolls using probiotic-packed ingredients. Use nori sheets as wraps and fill them with cooked brown rice, thinly sliced vegetables like cucumber and

avocado, and fermented ingredients like pickled ginger or kimchi. Serve with a side of probiotic-rich miso soup.

Wholesome dinners for optimal gut health

Dinner is an opportunity to nourish your body with a wholesome meal that supports optimal gut health. Here are some ideas for creating dinners with probiotic components:

- Stir-Fry with Fermented Vegetables: Prepare a colorful stir-fry using a variety of vegetables like broccoli, bell peppers, carrots, and snap peas. Add fermented vegetables like sauerkraut or kimchi for probiotic benefits. Incorporate lean protein sources like tofu, shrimp, or chicken, and serve over brown rice or noodles.
- Grilled Fish with Probiotic Salsa: Grill a piece of fatty fish like salmon or mackerel and serve it with a homemade salsa made from probiotic-rich ingredients like fermented tomatoes, onions, garlic, and fresh herbs. Pair with a side of steamed vegetables or a quinoa salad.
- Quinoa-Stuffed Peppers with Yogurt Sauce: Prepare stuffed bell peppers by filling them with a mixture of cooked quinoa, sautéed vegetables, and fermented feta cheese. Bake until tender and serve with a side of probiotic-rich yogurt sauce made with herbs and spices.
- Lentil Curry with Fermented Pickles: Make a flavorful lentil curry using a combination of lentils, spices, and vegetables. Add fermented pickles for a probiotic twist. Serve the curry over

brown rice or with whole wheat naan bread for a satisfying and gut-friendly dinner.

By incorporating probiotic components into your balanced meals throughout the day, you can support your gut health and overall well-being. Remember to experiment with different ingredients and flavors to create a variety of delicious and nutritious meals.

The Probiotic Diet and Weight Management
How probiotics can support healthy weight loss

Probiotics, the beneficial bacteria found in certain foods and supplements, can play a role in supporting healthy weight loss. While they are not a magical solution for shedding pounds, incorporating probiotics into your diet can have several benefits that contribute to weight management. Here's how probiotics can support your weight loss journey:

- Improved Digestion: Probiotics aid in the breakdown and absorption of nutrients from the foods you eat. By optimizing digestion, they ensure that your body efficiently extracts essential nutrients, vitamins, and minerals. This can help prevent nutritional deficiencies and support overall health, which is crucial for sustainable weight loss.
- Enhanced Gut Health: Probiotics promote a healthy gut microbiota, the community of microorganisms in your digestive system. A balanced and diverse gut microbiota is associated with better weight management. It helps regulate metabolism, reduces inflammation, and supports healthy digestion, all of which are important

factors in achieving and maintaining a healthy weight.

- Appetite Regulation: Probiotics can influence appetite-regulating hormones such as leptin and ghrelin, which control hunger and satiety. Research suggests that certain strains of probiotics may help reduce appetite, increase feelings of fullness, and decrease food cravings. By managing your appetite, probiotics can support portion control and prevent overeating, leading to better weight management.
- Reduced Inflammation: Chronic inflammation in the body can contribute to weight gain and hinder weight loss efforts. Probiotics have been shown to reduce inflammation by modulating the immune response and promoting a healthy gut lining. By reducing inflammation, probiotics can create a favorable environment for weight loss and overall well-being.

Probiotic foods for appetite control and satiety

Incorporating probiotic-rich foods into your diet can aid in appetite control and promote satiety, helping you manage your calorie intake and support your weight loss goals. Here are some probiotic foods that can assist with appetite control:

- Greek Yogurt: Greek yogurt is a popular probiotic-rich food that is also high in protein. Protein is known to promote feelings of fullness and reduce appetite. Choose plain, unsweetened Greek yogurt to avoid added sugars and enhance its probiotic benefits. Add fresh fruits or a sprinkle of nuts for added flavor and texture.

- Kefir: Kefir is a fermented dairy product similar to yogurt but with a thinner consistency. It is packed with probiotics and can be enjoyed on its own or blended into smoothies for a creamy and tangy addition. The combination of probiotics and protein in kefir can help promote satiety and control cravings.
- Fermented Vegetables: Incorporating fermented vegetables like sauerkraut or kimchi into your meals can provide probiotics and a satisfying crunch. These probiotic-rich foods are low in calories and can be enjoyed as a side dish or added to salads, wraps, or Buddha bowls for extra flavor and appetite control.
- Tempeh: Tempeh is a fermented soy product that offers a good amount of probiotics along with plant-based protein. It can be used as a meat substitute in various dishes, such as stir-fries, sandwiches, or grain bowls. The combination of probiotics and protein in tempeh can contribute to feelings of fullness and help regulate appetite.

The role of probiotics in regulating metabolism

Probiotics can also play a role in regulating metabolism, which is the process by which your body converts food into energy. Here's how probiotics can impact metabolism and potentially support weight management:

- Gut Microbiota Influence: The gut microbiota, where probiotics reside, has a complex relationship with metabolism. A healthy and diverse gut microbiota is associated with a more efficient metabolism, while an imbalanced microbiota has been linked to metabolic disorders and weight gain. Probiotics can help maintain a balanced gut microbiota, promoting a healthy metabolism.

- Short-Chain Fatty Acids (SCFAs): Probiotics produce short-chain fatty acids (SCFAs) during the fermentation process in the gut. SCFAs, such as butyrate, have been shown to have beneficial effects on metabolism. They can improve insulin sensitivity, which is important for maintaining stable blood sugar levels and preventing weight gain.
- Energy Extraction: Probiotics aid in the breakdown and absorption of nutrients, ensuring that your body extracts energy efficiently from the foods you consume. This efficient energy extraction can help support a healthy metabolism and prevent excess energy from being stored as fat.
- Lipid Metabolism: Some studies suggest that certain strains of probiotics may influence lipid metabolism, which refers to how your body processes and utilizes fats. Probiotics can help regulate lipid metabolism, potentially leading to better fat utilization and weight management.

Creating a sustainable eating plan for weight management

When it comes to weight management, creating a sustainable eating plan is essential for long-term success. Here are some tips for developing a balanced and probiotic-rich eating plan:

- Include a Variety of Probiotic Foods: Incorporate a range of probiotic-rich foods into your diet to ensure you're getting different strains of beneficial bacteria. Experiment with options like yogurt, kefir, fermented vegetables, tempeh, and kombucha to diversify your probiotic intake.
- Prioritize Whole Foods: Build your meals around whole, unprocessed foods that provide a wide array of nutrients. Focus on incorporating fruits, vegetables, whole grains, lean proteins, and healthy fats into your eating plan. These nutrient-dense foods support overall health and weight management.
- Practice Portion Control: Be mindful of portion sizes to avoid overeating. Even with probiotic foods, it's important to maintain a calorie balance for weight management. Pay attention to your hunger and fullness cues, and aim for balanced meals that include protein, fiber, and healthy fats to promote satiety.
- Practice Mindful Eating: Slow down and savor your meals. Mindful eating involves being present and fully engaged with the eating experience. It can help you recognize your body's hunger and fullness signals, preventing mindless snacking and overeating.
- Stay Hydrated: Drinking an adequate amount of water throughout the day is important for overall health and can also support weight management. Hydration helps maintain proper digestion, nutrient absorption, and a healthy metabolism.
- Seek Professional Guidance: If you're looking to develop a personalized eating plan for

weight management, consider consulting with a registered dietitian or nutritionist. They can provide individualized guidance, help you incorporate probiotic-rich foods, and ensure your eating plan meets your specific nutritional needs.

Remember, sustainable weight management involves a holistic approach that includes regular physical activity, stress management, and adequate sleep in addition to a balanced eating plan. Probiotic foods can be a valuable component of this approach, supporting your weight loss efforts and overall well-being.

Exercise and Probiotics: Enhancing Performance and Recovery
How probiotics can improve exercise performance

Probiotics, the beneficial bacteria found in certain foods and supplements, have been gaining attention for their potential to improve exercise performance. While more research is needed, there is emerging evidence suggesting that probiotics can offer benefits for athletes and active individuals. Here's how probiotics may help enhance exercise performance:

- Enhanced Nutrient Absorption: Probiotics support optimal digestion and nutrient absorption, which is crucial for providing the body with the necessary fuel and nutrients during exercise. By improving nutrient uptake, probiotics can ensure that the body efficiently utilizes carbohydrates, proteins, and fats for energy production and muscle function.
- Reduced Gastrointestinal Distress: Intense exercise can sometimes lead to gastrointestinal

distress, including symptoms like bloating, cramping, and diarrhea. Probiotics have been shown to help alleviate these symptoms by promoting a healthy gut environment and improving gut barrier function. By reducing gastrointestinal distress, probiotics may improve exercise tolerance and performance.

- Immune System Support: Intense exercise can temporarily suppress the immune system, making athletes more susceptible to infections and illnesses. Probiotics can strengthen the immune system by modulating immune responses and promoting a balanced gut microbiota. By supporting immune function, probiotics may help athletes stay healthy and maintain consistent training.

- Mitigation of Oxidative Stress: Intense exercise can generate oxidative stress in the body, leading to muscle damage and fatigue. Probiotics have antioxidant properties and can help reduce oxidative stress, potentially improving exercise performance and enhancing recovery.

Probiotics for reducing exercise-induced inflammation

Exercise-induced inflammation is a natural response of the body to physical activity. While inflammation is a crucial part of the recovery process, excessive or prolonged inflammation can hinder performance and delay recovery. Probiotics may help modulate the inflammatory response, promoting a healthier balance. Here's how probiotics can contribute to reducing exercise-induced inflammation:

- Anti-inflammatory Effects: Certain strains

of probiotics, such as Lactobacillus and Bifidobacterium species, have demonstrated anti-inflammatory properties. They can help reduce the production of pro-inflammatory molecules and promote the release of anti-inflammatory compounds, thereby modulating the inflammatory response associated with exercise.

- Gut Barrier Integrity: Probiotics play a role in maintaining the integrity of the gut barrier. A compromised gut barrier can lead to the leakage of bacterial toxins into the bloodstream, triggering systemic inflammation. By promoting a healthy gut barrier, probiotics may help reduce exercise-induced inflammation.
- Regulation of Immune Responses: Probiotics can influence immune responses, including the production of inflammatory cytokines. By modulating immune activity, probiotics may help regulate the inflammatory response to exercise and prevent excessive inflammation.
- Reduction of Oxidative Stress: Exercise-induced inflammation is often accompanied by oxidative stress. Probiotics possess antioxidant properties and can help neutralize free radicals, reducing oxidative stress and its associated inflammation.

The role of gut health in post-exercise recovery

Post-exercise recovery is crucial for repairing muscles, replenishing energy stores, and adapting to exercise. Gut health plays a significant role in the recovery process. Here's how a healthy gut can contribute to post-exercise recovery:

- Nutrient Absorption: A healthy gut microbiota aids in the efficient absorption of nutrients, including carbohydrates, proteins, and micronutrients. After exercise, the body requires these nutrients for muscle repair, glycogen replenishment, and overall recovery. Probiotics promote a balanced gut environment, optimizing nutrient absorption and supporting post-exercise recovery.
- Immune Function: Intense exercise can temporarily suppress the immune system, increasing the risk of infections and compromising recovery. The gut is a major site of immune activity, and a healthy gut microbiota helps support immune function. By promoting a diverse and balanced gut microbiota, probiotics can enhance immune responses and facilitate faster recovery.
- Gut Barrier Integrity: Exercise-induced stress and inflammation can affect the integrity of the gut barrier. A compromised gut barrier allows harmful substances to leak into the bloodstream, triggering inflammation and delaying recovery. Probiotics help maintain the integrity of the gut barrier, reducing the risk of leakage and promoting a healthy recovery process.
- Reduction of Gastrointestinal Distress: Gastrointestinal symptoms, such as bloating, cramping, and diarrhea, can interfere with post-exercise recovery. Probiotics have been shown to alleviate gastrointestinal distress by improving gut function and reducing inflammation. By minimizing these symptoms, probiotics

contribute to a smoother and more efficient recovery process.

Incorporating probiotics into your fitness routine

To incorporate probiotics into your fitness routine, consider the following strategies:

- Probiotic Supplements: Probiotic supplements are available in various forms, such as capsules, tablets, powders, and liquids. Choose a high-quality probiotic supplement with strains that are known to support gut health and exercise performance. Follow the recommended dosage instructions provided by the manufacturer or consult with a healthcare professional.
- Probiotic-Rich Foods: Include probiotic-rich foods in your diet to naturally boost your probiotic intake. Examples of probiotic-rich foods include yogurt, kefir, sauerkraut, kimchi, kombucha, and miso. Be sure to choose varieties that contain live and active cultures for maximum probiotic benefits.
- Timing: Consider the timing of your probiotic intake to optimize its effects. Consuming probiotics before or after exercise may be beneficial for supporting gut health and recovery. Experiment with different timing strategies to find what works best for you.
- Balanced Diet: Support the growth and diversity of beneficial gut bacteria by maintaining a balanced and nutritious diet. Include fiber-rich foods, such as fruits, vegetables, whole grains, and legumes, as they serve as prebiotics, which

nourish the probiotic bacteria in your gut.

- Monitor Your Response: Pay attention to how your body responds to probiotics. Everyone's digestive system is unique, and some individuals may experience temporary changes in digestion when introducing probiotics. Monitor any effects and adjust your probiotic intake or strain selection accordingly.

- Seek Professional Advice: If you have specific concerns or conditions related to gut health or exercise performance, it's advisable to consult with a healthcare professional, such as a registered dietitian or sports nutritionist. They can provide personalized recommendations based on your individual needs and goals.

Remember that while probiotics may offer potential benefits for exercise performance and recovery, they should be seen as a complement to a well-rounded fitness routine, including proper nutrition, hydration, rest, and appropriate training protocols.

CHAPTER TWO

Greek Yogurt Bowl

Description: This refreshing Greek Yogurt Bowl is a delightful combination of creamy yogurt, vibrant fresh berries, crunchy nuts, and a sweet drizzle of honey. It's a perfect balance of flavors and textures that will leave you feeling satisfied and energized.

Ingredients:

- 1 cup Greek yogurt
- Assorted fresh berries (strawberries, blueberries, raspberries)
- Handful of mixed nuts (almonds, walnuts, cashews)
- Drizzle of honey

Instructions:

- In a bowl, scoop the Greek yogurt as a base.
- Arrange the fresh berries on top of the yogurt.
- Sprinkle the mixed nuts over the berries.
- Finish off by drizzling a generous amount of honey over the bowl.
- Mix everything together before enjoying this delicious and nutritious Greek Yogurt Bowl.

Nutritional Information:

Calories: 250

Protein: 15g

Carbohydrates: 25g

Fat: 10g

Fiber: 5g

Kimchi Fried Rice

Description: Kimchi Fried Rice is a flavorful and satisfying dish that combines the tangy goodness of fermented kimchi with wholesome brown rice and a medley of mixed vegetables. It's a perfect balance of umami and spice, making it a great choice for a quick and tasty meal.

Ingredients:

- 2 cups cooked brown rice
- 1 cup fermented kimchi, chopped
- Assorted mixed vegetables (carrots, bell peppers, peas, corn)
- 2 tablespoons soy sauce
- 1 tablespoon sesame oil
- 2 green onions, chopped
- Sesame seeds for garnish

Instructions:

- Heat a tablespoon of oil in a large skillet or wok over medium heat.
- Add the mixed vegetables and sauté until they are slightly tender.
- Stir in the chopped kimchi and cook for a few more minutes.
- Add the cooked brown rice to the skillet and mix well with the vegetables and kimchi.
- Drizzle soy sauce and sesame oil over the rice mixture and stir to combine.
- Cook for an additional 5 minutes, stirring occasionally, until the flavors meld together.

- Garnish with chopped green onions and sprinkle sesame seeds on top.
- Serve hot and enjoy the deliciousness of Kimchi Fried Rice!

Nutritional Information:

Calories: 350

Protein: 10g

Carbohydrates: 50g

Fat: 8g

Fiber: 7g

Grilled Chicken Breast

Description: Grilled Chicken Breast is a simple and nutritious meal that features tender and juicy chicken breast served alongside tangy sauerkraut and a side of steamed vegetables. It's a protein-packed dish that will satisfy your taste buds and keep you feeling full and satisfied.

Ingredients:

- 2 boneless, skinless chicken breasts
- Salt and pepper to taste
- 1 cup sauerkraut
- Assorted steamed vegetables (broccoli, cauliflower, carrots)

Instructions:

- Preheat the grill to medium-high heat.
- Season the chicken breasts with salt and pepper on both sides.
- Place the chicken on the grill and cook for

about 6-8 minutes per side, or until the internal temperature reaches 165°F (74°C).

- Remove the chicken from the grill and let it rest for a few minutes before slicing.
- Serve the grilled chicken breast with a side of sauerkraut and steamed vegetables.
- Enjoy the flavorful combination of grilled chicken, tangy sauerkraut, and nutritious vegetables!

Nutritional Information:

Calories: 300

Protein: 40g

Carbohydrates: 10g

Fat: 8g

Fiber: 5g

Quinoa Salad

Description: Quinoa Salad is a vibrant and refreshing dish that combines the nutty flavors of quinoa with a mix of fermented vegetables like pickles, beets, and carrots. It's a colorful and satisfying salad that provides a great combination of textures and flavors.

Ingredients:

- 1 cup cooked quinoa
- Assorted fermented vegetables (pickles, beets, carrots), chopped
- Handful of fresh herbs (parsley, cilantro), chopped
- Juice of 1 lemon
- 2 tablespoons olive oil
- Salt and pepper to taste

Instructions:

- In a large bowl, combine the cooked quinoa, fermented vegetables, and fresh herbs.
- In a separate small bowl, whisk together the lemon juice, olive oil, salt, and pepper to make the dressing.
- Pour the dressing over the quinoa mixture and toss well to combine.
- Adjust the seasoning if needed.
- Allow the flavors to meld together for about 10 minutes before serving.
- Serve the Quinoa Salad as a refreshing and nutritious side dish or a light meal.

Nutritional Information:

Calories: 200

Protein: 6g

Carbohydrates: 30g

Fat: 7g

Fiber: 5g

Tempeh Stir-Fry

Description: Tempeh Stir-Fry is a flavorful and nutritious dish that combines protein-rich tempeh with vibrant broccoli, bell peppers, and a zesty ginger-garlic sauce. It's a satisfying and wholesome meal that will tantalize your taste buds and provide a good dose of plant-based goodness.

Ingredients:

- 8 oz tempeh, cubed
- 2 cups broccoli florets

- 1 bell pepper, sliced
- 2 cloves garlic, minced
- 1 tablespoon fresh ginger, grated
- 2 tablespoons soy sauce
- 1 tablespoon maple syrup
- 1 tablespoon rice vinegar
- 1 tablespoon sesame oil
- 2 green onions, chopped
- Sesame seeds for garnish
- Cooked rice or noodles (optional)

Instructions:

- In a large skillet or wok, heat sesame oil over medium heat.
- Add the tempeh cubes and cook until lightly browned and crispy on all sides.
- Remove the tempeh from the skillet and set aside.
- In the same skillet, add the garlic and ginger, and sauté for a minute until fragrant.
- Add the broccoli florets and bell pepper slices, and stir-fry for about 5 minutes until tender-crisp.
- In a small bowl, whisk together soy sauce, maple syrup, and rice vinegar to make the sauce.
- Pour the sauce into the skillet and add the cooked tempeh.
- Stir-fry everything together for another 2-3 minutes until the sauce coats the vegetables and tempeh.
- Remove from heat and garnish with chopped green onions and sesame seeds.
- Serve the Tempeh Stir-Fry as is or over cooked rice or noodles for a complete meal.

Nutritional Information:

Calories: 350

Protein: 20g

Carbohydrates: 30g

Fat: 16g

Fiber: 8g

Miso Soup

Description: Miso Soup is a comforting and nourishing Japanese soup that combines umami-rich miso paste with tofu, seaweed, and green onions. It's a light yet satisfying soup that is packed with flavor and provides a healthy dose of nutrients.

Ingredients:

- 4 cups vegetable broth
- 3 tablespoons miso paste
- 1 cup firm tofu, cubed
- 1/4 cup dried seaweed (such as wakame or kombu), rehydrated
- 2 green onions, sliced

Instructions:

- In a pot, bring the vegetable broth to a gentle simmer over medium heat.
- In a small bowl, whisk together the miso paste with a small amount of hot broth to dissolve it.
- Add the dissolved miso paste, tofu cubes, and rehydrated seaweed to the pot.
- Simmer for 5 minutes, stirring occasionally.
- Taste and adjust the seasoning, adding more miso paste if desired.
- Remove from heat and garnish with sliced green

onions.

- Serve the Miso Soup hot and enjoy its comforting and nutritious qualities.

Nutritional Information:

Calories: 120

Protein: 8g

Carbohydrates: 12g

Fat: 5g

Fiber: 3g

Probiotic Smoothie

Description: This Probiotic Smoothie is a refreshing and healthy blend of kefir, spinach, banana, and flaxseeds. It's a delicious way to boost your gut health and provide your body with essential nutrients.

Ingredients:

- 1 cup kefir
- Handful of fresh spinach leaves
- 1 ripe banana
- 1 tablespoon flaxseeds

Instructions:

- In a blender, combine kefir, spinach, banana, and flaxseeds.
- Blend on high speed until smooth and creamy.
- If the smoothie is too thick, you can add a splash of water or more kefir to achieve the desired consistency.
- Pour into a glass and enjoy this Probiotic Smoothie as a nutritious breakfast or snack.

Nutritional Information:

Calories: 200

Protein: 10g

Carbohydrates: 35g

Fat: 5g

Fiber: 8g

Fermented Vegetable Wrap

Description: The Fermented Vegetable Wrap is a delightful combination of tangy fermented vegetables, creamy hummus, ripe avocado, and fresh sprouts. It's a colorful and flavorful wrap that is not only delicious but also packed with beneficial probiotics and nutrients.

Ingredients:

- Large whole-grain tortilla or wrap
- 1/4 cup fermented vegetables (such as sauerkraut or kimchi)
- 2 tablespoons hummus
- 1/2 ripe avocado, sliced
- Handful of fresh sprouts (such as alfalfa or broccoli sprouts)

Instructions:

- Lay the tortilla or wrap on a flat surface.
- Spread hummus evenly over the surface of the wrap.
- Place fermented vegetables, avocado slices, and sprouts in the center of the wrap.
- Carefully roll the wrap, tucking in the sides as you go, until it is tightly sealed.
- Slice the wrap in half, if desired, for easier

handling.

- Enjoy the Fermented Vegetable Wrap as a nutritious and flavorful meal or snack.

Nutritional Information:

Calories: 300

Protein: 8g

Carbohydrates: 40g

Fat: 15g

Fiber: 10g

Baked Salmon

Description: Baked Salmon is a flavorful and nutritious dish that features tender and flaky salmon fillets baked to perfection. It is served with a refreshing yogurt-based cucumber salad that complements the richness of the salmon. This meal is packed with omega-3 fatty acids, protein, and probiotics.

Ingredients:

- 2 salmon fillets
- Salt and pepper to taste
- 1 lemon, sliced
- 1 cucumber, thinly sliced
- 1 cup Greek yogurt
- 1 tablespoon fresh dill, chopped
- 1 tablespoon fresh lemon juice
- 1 tablespoon extra-virgin olive oil

Instructions:

- Preheat the oven to 375°F (190°C).
- Season the salmon fillets with salt and pepper

and place them on a baking sheet lined with parchment paper.

- Top each fillet with a couple of lemon slices.
- Bake the salmon for 12-15 minutes or until it is cooked through and flakes easily with a fork.
- While the salmon is baking, prepare the cucumber salad by combining sliced cucumber, Greek yogurt, fresh dill, lemon juice, and olive oil in a bowl.
- Season the cucumber salad with salt and pepper to taste and mix well.
- Once the salmon is cooked, serve it with a side of the refreshing yogurt-based cucumber salad.
- Enjoy the delicious and nutritious Baked Salmon with Cucumber Salad.

Nutritional Information:

Calories: 350

Protein: 30g

Carbohydrates: 10g

Fat: 20g

Fiber: 2g

Probiotic-Rich Salad

Description: The Probiotic-Rich Salad is a vibrant and nutritious mix of mixed greens, fermented vegetables, and a zesty lemon-tahini dressing. This salad is loaded with probiotics, vitamins, and minerals, making it a perfect choice for a healthy and refreshing meal.

Ingredients:

- 4 cups mixed greens (spinach, arugula, kale)

- 1 cup fermented vegetables (such as sauerkraut or kimchi)
- 1/2 cup cherry tomatoes, halved
- 1/4 cup sliced cucumber
- 1/4 cup sliced radishes
- 2 tablespoons tahini
- Juice of 1 lemon
- 2 tablespoons extra-virgin olive oil
- Salt and pepper to taste

Instructions:

- In a large salad bowl, combine the mixed greens, fermented vegetables, cherry tomatoes, sliced cucumber, and sliced radishes.
- In a separate small bowl, whisk together tahini, lemon juice, olive oil, salt, and pepper to make the dressing.
- Pour the dressing over the salad and toss well to coat the ingredients evenly.
- Adjust the seasoning if needed.
- Serve the Probiotic-Rich Salad as a refreshing and nutritious meal or side dish.

Nutritional Information:

Calories: 200

Protein: 5g

Carbohydrates: 15g

Fat: 15g

Fiber: 5g

Black Bean and Sauerkraut Tacos

Description: Black Bean and Sauerkraut Tacos are a

delightful fusion of flavors and textures. The combination of hearty black beans, tangy sauerkraut, and a dollop of creamy Greek yogurt creates a satisfying and probiotic-rich meal.

Ingredients:

- 8 small corn tortillas
- 1 can black beans, rinsed and drained
- 1 cup sauerkraut
- 1/2 cup Greek yogurt
- 1/4 cup fresh cilantro, chopped
- Lime wedges for serving

Instructions:

- Warm the corn tortillas on a dry skillet over medium heat until soft and pliable.
- In a small saucepan, heat the black beans over medium heat until heated through.
- Assemble the tacos by layering the warm tortillas with a spoonful of black beans, a generous amount of sauerkraut, a dollop of Greek yogurt, and a sprinkle of fresh cilantro.
- Squeeze fresh lime juice over the tacos for added zest.
- Serve the Black Bean and Sauerkraut Tacos as a flavorful and probiotic-packed meal.

Nutritional Information:

Calories: 250

Protein: 10g

Carbohydrates: 40g

Fat: 4g

Fiber: 10g

Probiotic Bowl

Description: The Probiotic Bowl is a nourishing and satisfying meal that combines cooked quinoa, protein-rich tempeh, tangy fermented beets, and creamy sliced avocado. This bowl is not only delicious but also provides a good balance of nutrients and probiotics.

Ingredients:

- 1 cup cooked quinoa
- 8 oz tempeh, cubed and cooked
- 1/2 cup fermented beets, chopped
- 1 ripe avocado, sliced
- Handful of fresh greens (such as spinach or kale)
- 2 tablespoons lemon-tahini dressing (from the Probiotic-Rich Salad recipe)

Instructions:

- In a bowl, arrange the cooked quinoa, cooked tempeh, fermented beets, sliced avocado, and fresh greens.
- Drizzle the lemon-tahini dressing over the ingredients.
- Toss gently to combine all the elements.
- Serve the Probiotic Bowl as a nourishing and flavorful meal.

Nutritional Information:

Calories: 400

Protein: 20g

Carbohydrates: 40g

Fat: 20g

Fiber: 10g

Lentil Soup

Description: Lentil Soup is a comforting and nutritious dish made with protein-packed lentils, flavorful vegetables, and warming spices. To enhance its probiotic content, it is served with a dollop of probiotic-rich yogurt or kefir. This soup is hearty, filling, and packed with beneficial nutrients.

Ingredients:

- 1 cup dried lentils, rinsed and drained
- 1 onion, diced
- 2 carrots, diced
- 2 celery stalks, diced
- 3 cloves garlic, minced
- 4 cups vegetable broth
- 1 teaspoon ground cumin
- 1 teaspoon ground turmeric
- 1/2 teaspoon ground paprika
- Salt and pepper to taste
- Probiotic-rich yogurt or kefir for serving

Instructions:

- In a large pot, heat some oil over medium heat.
- Add the diced onion, carrots, celery, and minced garlic to the pot. Sauté until the vegetables are tender.
- Add the lentils, vegetable broth, cumin, turmeric, and paprika to the pot. Stir well to combine.
- Bring the mixture to a boil, then reduce the heat and let it simmer for about 25-30 minutes, or until the lentils are cooked and tender.
- Season with salt and pepper to taste.
- Ladle the lentil soup into bowls and top each serving with a dollop of probiotic-rich yogurt or

kefir.

- Enjoy this comforting Lentil Soup with the added goodness of probiotics.

Nutritional Information:

Calories: 250

Protein: 15g

Carbohydrates: 40g

Fat: 2g

Fiber: 15g

Fermented Vegetable and Tofu Stir-Fry

Description: Fermented Vegetable and Tofu Stir-Fry is a flavorful and probiotic-rich dish that combines tangy fermented vegetables, protein-packed tofu, and nutritious brown rice noodles. This stir-fry is a wholesome and satisfying meal that can be easily prepared in no time.

Ingredients:

- 8 oz brown rice noodles, cooked according to package instructions
- 8 oz firm tofu, drained and cubed
- 1 cup fermented vegetables (such as kimchi or sauerkraut)
- 1 bell pepper, sliced
- 1 small onion, sliced
- 3 cloves garlic, minced
- 2 tablespoons soy sauce
- 1 tablespoon sesame oil
- Sesame seeds for garnish

Instructions:

- In a large skillet or wok, heat sesame oil over medium heat.
- Add the cubed tofu and sauté until lightly browned and crispy on all sides. Remove from the skillet and set aside.
- In the same skillet, add the minced garlic, sliced bell pepper, and onion. Stir-fry for a few minutes until the vegetables are tender-crisp.
- Add the cooked brown rice noodles, fermented vegetables, and sautéed tofu to the skillet.
- Drizzle soy sauce over the ingredients and toss everything together to combine well.
- Continue stir-frying for a few more minutes until everything is heated through.
- Remove from heat and garnish with sesame seeds.
- Serve the Fermented Vegetable and Tofu Stir-Fry as a delicious and probiotic-packed meal.

Nutritional Information:

Calories: 400

Protein: 15g

Carbohydrates: 60g

Fat: 10g

Fiber: 8g

Probiotic Smoothie Bowl

Description: The Probiotic Smoothie Bowl is a refreshing and nutritious treat that combines the goodness of probiotics, fruits, and seeds. It is a vibrant and filling breakfast option that will leave you energized and satisfied. Top it with granola, sliced fruit, and a sprinkle of chia seeds for added texture and flavor.

Ingredients:

- 1 cup probiotic-rich yogurt or kefir
- 1 ripe banana
- 1 cup frozen berries (such as blueberries or strawberries)
- 1 tablespoon flaxseeds
- Granola for topping
- Sliced fruit (such as kiwi or berries) for topping
- Chia seeds for sprinkling

Instructions:

- In a blender, combine the probiotic-rich yogurt or kefir, ripe banana, frozen berries, and flaxseeds.
- Blend on high speed until smooth and creamy.
- Pour the smoothie into a bowl.
- Top with granola, sliced fruit, and a sprinkle of chia seeds.
- Serve the Probiotic Smoothie Bowl immediately and enjoy this nourishing and delightful breakfast option.

Nutritional Information:

Calories: 300

Protein: 15g

Carbohydrates: 45g

Fat: 8g

Fiber: 10g

CONCLUSION

In conclusion, the probiotic diet offers a compelling and scientifically-backed approach to improving our overall health and well-being. By harnessing the power of beneficial bacteria, we have the opportunity to optimize our digestion, strengthen our immune system, and promote a healthy balance within our bodies. Throughout this book, we have explored the profound impact of probiotics on various aspects of our health, from gut health and weight management to mental well-being and skin health. We have learned about the different types of probiotics, their food sources, and the best practices for incorporating them into our daily lives.

As we close this chapter, it is important to emphasize that the probiotic diet is not a one-size-fits-all solution. Each of us has a unique microbiome, and what works for one person may not yield the same results for another. It is essential to listen to our bodies, experiment with different probiotic-rich foods, and consult with healthcare professionals when necessary.

The journey towards optimal health is ongoing, and embracing a probiotic-rich lifestyle is a lifelong commitment. By nourishing our bodies with beneficial bacteria and making conscious choices about our diet and lifestyle, we can cultivate a harmonious relationship with our microbiome and unlock the potential for enhanced vitality and well-being.

May this book serve as a guide and source of inspiration

on your probiotic journey. Here's to a healthier, happier you, empowered by the transformative power of probiotics. Cheers to a vibrant and thriving life!

www.ingramcontent.com/pod-product-compliance
Lightning Source LLC
Chambersburg PA
CBHW070046260726
48658CB00002B/757